Methylene Blue

A Beginner's Quick Start Guide on Its Use Cases, Applications, and Benefits, with Answers to Common Questions copyright © 2024 Tyler Spellmann

All rights reserved No part of this book may be reproduced, or stored in a retrieval system, or transmitted in any form or by any means, electronic, mechanical, photocopying, recording, or otherwise, without express written permission of the publisher.

Disclaimer

By reading this disclaimer, you are accepting the terms of the disclaimer in full. If you disagree with this disclaimer, please do not read the guide.

All of the content within this guide is provided for informational and educational purposes only, and should not be accepted as independent medical or other professional advice. The author is not a doctor, physician, nurse, mental health provider, or registered nutritionist/dietician. Therefore, using and reading this guide does not establish any form of a physician-patient relationship.

Always consult with a physician or another qualified health provider with any issues or questions you might have regarding any sort of medical condition. Do not ever disregard any qualified professional medical advice or delay seeking that advice because of anything you have read in this guide. The information in this guide is not intended to be any sort of medical advice and should not be used in lieu of any medical advice by a licensed and qualified medical professional.

The information in this guide has been compiled from a variety of known sources. However, the author cannot attest to or guarantee the accuracy of each source and thus should not be held liable for any errors or omissions.

You acknowledge that the publisher of this guide will not be held liable for any loss or damage of any kind incurred as a result of this guide or the reliance on any information provided within this guide. You acknowledge and agree that you assume all risk and responsibility for any action you undertake in response to the information in this guide.

Using this guide does not guarantee any particular result (e.g., weight loss or a cure). By reading this guide, you acknowledge that there are no guarantees to any specific outcome or results you can expect.

All product names, diet plans, or names used in this guide are for identification purposes only and are the property of their respective owners. The use of these names does not imply endorsement. All other trademarks cited herein are the property of their respective owners.

Where applicable, this guide is not intended to be a substitute for the original work of this diet plan and is, at most, a supplement to the original work for this diet plan and never a direct substitute. This guide is a personal expression of the facts of that diet plan.

Where applicable, persons shown in the cover images are stock photography models and the publisher has obtained the rights to use the images through license agreements with third-party stock image companies.

Table of Contents

Introduction	6
What Is Methylene Blue?	8
Chemical Composition and Properties	9
How does Methylene Blue Work?	10
Use Cases of Methylene Blue	15
Medical Applications	15
Industrial Uses	18
Veterinary Medicine	21
Ongoing Research and Development	23
Health Benefits of the Methylene Blue	23
Disadvantages of the Methylene Blue	25
Pros and Cons of the Methylene Blue Treatment	30
Pros	30
Cons	33
A Step-by-step Guide to Understanding Methylene Blue	36
Step 1: Educate Yourself on the Proper Usage of Methylene Blue	36
Step 2: Recognize Potential Side Effects	41
Step 3: Implement Safety Precautions	44
Step 4: Monitor Your Health	48
Step 5: Understand Long-term Use Implications	53
Step 6: Know When to Seek Help	59
Potential Side Effects	63
Contraindications and Precautions	71
Guidelines for Safe Usage	75
Conclusion	78
FAQs	82
References and Helpful Links	85

Introduction

Methylene Blue stands as a pivotal compound in numerous fields, owing to its diverse applications and benefits. In the medical sector, it is renowned for its therapeutic properties, notably in the treatment of methemoglobinemia—a condition affecting oxygen delivery in the body. Additionally, its diagnostic utility as a staining agent is invaluable, facilitating detailed visualization of cellular components in scientific research.

The compound's versatility extends beyond healthcare. In the textile industry, it continues to be used to impart color to fabrics. Meanwhile, its role as a redox agent in scientific studies has sparked interest in its potential for neuroprotection and cognitive enhancement. Researchers are actively exploring its effects on mitochondrial function and its implications for brain health, pointing to promising developments in addressing cognitive decline.

Nonetheless, the application of Methylene Blue comes with important considerations. It comes with a set of pros and cons that must be weighed to ensure safe and effective application.

Understanding these aspects is crucial for anyone looking to maximize its potential benefits while minimizing risks.

In this guide, we will talk about the following:

- What is Methylene Blue?
- Use Cases of Methylene Blue
- Pros and Cons of The Methylene Blue Treatment
- A Step-by-step Guide to Methylene Blue
- Potential Side Effects
- Contraindications and Precautions

Keep reading to discover more about this versatile compound and how it could potentially benefit you. By the end of this guide, you will have a better understanding of the potential applications of Methylene Blue and how you can use it safely and effectively in your personal or professional endeavors.

What Is Methylene Blue?

Methylene blue, a synthetic dye, was first discovered by German chemist Heinrich Caro in 1876. Initially, its vibrant blue coloration made it popular as a textile dye, marking its entry into industrial use. However, its potential extended far beyond coloring fabrics, leading to significant interest in its chemical properties and broader applications.

In the late 19th and early 20th centuries, methylene blue began to find its place in the medical field. It was introduced as an antiseptic and antibacterial agent, and by 1891, it became one of the first synthetic drugs used to treat malaria. This marked a pivotal point in its application, showcasing its potential in therapeutic contexts.

During the mid-20th century, methylene blue's role expanded further in the realm of medical diagnostics and treatment. It was utilized as a staining agent in various laboratory procedures, aiding in the visualization of cells and tissues under a microscope. Its application in methemoglobinemia treatment—where it acts as an antidote to correct abnormal hemoglobin levels—further solidified its medical relevance.

As research progressed, methylene blue found new applications in scientific research and industrial processes. It became a tool in neuroscience for tracking brain activities, owing to its ability to penetrate cell membranes and highlight neural pathways. Industrially, it was employed in water treatment processes to remove contaminants, benefiting from its chemical reactivity.

Today, methylene blue continues to evolve, with ongoing studies exploring its potential in areas such as photodynamic therapy and neuroprotection. Its journey from a simple dye to a compound with multifaceted applications reflects its dynamic adaptability and enduring importance across multiple fields.

Chemical Composition and Properties

Methylene blue, scientifically known as methylthioninium chloride, is a synthetic compound characterized by its distinctive chemical structure. At its core, it features a phenothiazine ring system — a tricyclic structure comprising three rings — linked to a thiazine group. This arrangement is crucial to its deep blue coloration and reactive properties. The chemical formula, $C_{16}H_{18}N_3SCl$, highlights its composition of carbon, hydrogen, nitrogen, sulfur, and chlorine atoms.

Physically, methylene blue appears as a dark green crystalline powder. When dissolved in water, it produces a vibrant blue solution due to its chromophore system, which absorbs light at specific wavelengths. This property makes it valuable in staining and diagnostic applications.

Chemically, methylene blue is an organic chloride salt with notable reactive tendencies. It acts as a redox indicator, capable of reversible reduction and oxidation. In its oxidized form, it retains its blue color, while reduction can lead to a colorless leucomethylene blue. This redox behavior is particularly useful in medical treatments for methemoglobinemia, where it converts methemoglobin back to hemoglobin.

Furthermore, methylene blue is soluble in water and ethanol, enhancing its versatility in scientific and industrial processes. Its stability under normal conditions and its ability to bind with various biological structures increase its utility in laboratory and medical settings.

The unique chemical composition and properties of methylene blue not only define its vibrant appearance but also underpin its adaptability and functionality across various domains.

How does Methylene Blue Work?

Methylene Blue is a versatile compound with a range of physiological effects, making it a valuable therapeutic agent in specific medical conditions. This section delves into the mechanisms through which Methylene Blue operates within the body, highlighting its primary roles and broader implications.

1. **Role in Converting Methemoglobin to Hemoglobin**

   Mechanism of Action

   - *Reducing Agent*: Methylene Blue functions as a reducing agent, meaning it donates electrons to other molecules. In the context of blood chemistry, it specifically targets methemoglobin, the oxidized form of hemoglobin. Methemoglobin contains ferric iron (Fe^{3+}) rather than the usual ferrous iron (Fe^{2+}), which impairs its ability to bind and release oxygen.
   - *Conversion Process*: By converting methemoglobin back into hemoglobin, Methylene Blue restores the hemoglobin's functionality, enabling red blood cells to efficiently carry and deliver oxygen throughout the body. This conversion is crucial in conditions like methemoglobinemia, where elevated levels of methemoglobin lead to reduced oxygen delivery to tissues.

2. **Treatment of Methemoglobinemia**

   Clinical Application

- *Methemoglobinemia Management*: Methylene Blue is particularly effective in treating methemoglobinemia, a condition characterized by increased levels of methemoglobin in the blood. This condition can arise from genetic disorders, exposure to certain drugs, or chemical agents.
- *Therapeutic Use*: As an antidote, Methylene Blue is administered intravenously to patients, rapidly reducing methemoglobin levels and alleviating symptoms such as cyanosis, fatigue, and shortness of breath. This treatment significantly improves oxygen transport and overall patient outcomes.

3. Effects on Smooth Muscle Contraction

Inhibition of Guanylate Cyclase

- *Guanylate Cyclase Inhibition*: Beyond its role in blood chemistry, Methylene Blue also affects smooth muscle function. It inhibits the enzyme guanylate cyclase, which is involved in the synthesis of cyclic guanosine monophosphate (cGMP). cGMP is a secondary messenger that mediates various physiological processes, including smooth muscle relaxation.
- *Impact on Vascular Tone*: By inhibiting guanylate cyclase, Methylene Blue can induce

smooth muscle contraction, affecting the tone of blood vessels and other smooth muscle tissues. This action may have implications in managing conditions where modulation of vascular tone is required.

4. **Broader Implications and Therapeutic Applications**
   Physiological Impact

   - *Oxygen Delivery*: The ability of Methylene Blue to restore hemoglobin's oxygen-carrying capacity has profound implications for treating conditions where oxygen delivery is compromised. It underscores the importance of maintaining optimal hemoglobin function for overall health.
   - *Vascular Effects*: The impact on smooth muscle contraction suggests potential therapeutic applications in cardiovascular medicine, where controlling vascular tone is crucial for managing blood pressure and blood flow.

Methylene Blue's dual role as a reducing agent and guanylate cyclase inhibitor highlights its therapeutic versatility. Its primary application in treating methemoglobinemia showcases its critical impact on oxygen transport, while its effects on smooth muscle contraction open avenues for broader clinical use. Understanding these mechanisms allows for the effective utilization of Methylene Blue in medical practice, enhancing patient care and treatment outcomes.

Use Cases of Methylene Blue

Methylene blue has been used in various fields and industries due to its diverse properties. Here are some notable use cases of this versatile chemical:

Medical Applications

Methylene blue has become a cornerstone in the medical field, largely due to its versatile applications and proven effectiveness in various treatments and procedures.

1. **Treatment of Methemoglobinemia**

    One of the primary medical uses of methylene blue is in the treatment of methemoglobinemia, a disorder characterized by elevated levels of methemoglobin, a form of hemoglobin that cannot bind oxygen efficiently. This condition can lead to hypoxia and cyanosis. Methylene blue works by serving as an artificial electron carrier, facilitating the conversion of methemoglobin back to hemoglobin through the NADPH-dependent methemoglobin reductase pathway.

The treatment is notably quick, with patients often experiencing relief from symptoms shortly after administration. Its efficacy has made it a standard emergency treatment in cases of drug-induced or congenital methemoglobinemia.

2. **Surgical Dye and Diagnostic Tool**

In surgery, methylene blue is invaluable for its role as a visual aid. Surgeons frequently use it to stain tissues, which enhances visibility and precision during operations. This is particularly important in procedures such as sentinel lymph node biopsies in cancer surgeries, where methylene blue helps identify nodes that are likely to contain cancer cells, thus aiding in accurate staging and treatment planning. Additionally, its application extends to diagnostics, as it is used to detect fistulas or leaks in gastrointestinal and urinary tracts, where the dye's vivid color marks abnormal passages or breaks.

3. **Photodynamic Therapy**

Methylene blue's photodynamic properties make it suitable for photodynamic therapy (PDT), a treatment that combines a photosensitizing agent with light exposure to produce reactive oxygen species that can damage and kill cancer cells. This approach is gaining traction in oncology, particularly for superficial tumors and certain non-cancerous conditions.

Methylene blue is activated by specific wavelengths of light, leading to targeted cytotoxic effects that spare surrounding healthy tissues, making it a potentially safer alternative to more invasive treatments.

4. Neuroprotective Effects and Alzheimer's Disease

Recent research has brought attention to the neuroprotective potential of methylene blue. Studies suggest that it can mitigate oxidative stress and reduce inflammation, both of which are implicated in the progression of Alzheimer's disease.

By inhibiting tau protein aggregation, a hallmark of Alzheimer's, methylene blue may slow disease progression and improve cognitive function. Ongoing clinical trials are exploring its efficacy and safety in this context, with early results indicating a promising therapeutic role.

5. Additional Therapeutic Uses

Beyond its established applications, methylene blue is being investigated for other therapeutic uses. Its antimicrobial properties could be harnessed to treat infections resistant to conventional antibiotics.

Moreover, its ability to cross the blood-brain barrier and modulate mitochondrial function is being studied for potential benefits in other neurodegenerative disorders and conditions associated with mitochondrial dysfunction.

In summary, methylene blue's diverse applications in medicine highlight its importance as both a therapeutic and diagnostic agent. While its established uses continue to benefit patients, ongoing research is likely to expand its role, potentially offering new treatment avenues for a variety of conditions.

Industrial Uses

Methylene blue serves a variety of crucial roles in industrial applications, leveraging its chemical properties to enhance processes across multiple sectors.

1. **Role as a Redox Indicator**

   Methylene blue is widely used as a redox indicator in various industrial processes. Its ability to undergo reversible oxidation-reduction reactions makes it an essential tool for indicating the endpoint of chemical reactions.

   This feature is particularly valuable in industries like chemical manufacturing and environmental monitoring, where precise control over chemical processes is crucial. In redox reactions, methylene blue changes color from blue to colorless as it is reduced, providing a clear visual cue for reaction progress and completion.

2. Application in Paints, Inks, and Plastics Production

In the production of paints, inks, and plastics, methylene blue is utilized to monitor contamination levels and ensure the quality of the final product. Its sensitivity to changes in the chemical environment allows manufacturers to detect impurities and prevent defects that could compromise product integrity.

Moreover, as a dye, methylene blue can contribute to achieving specific hues in colored products, enhancing the aesthetic quality of paints and inks.

3. Antioxidant Additives in Fuels

As an antioxidant additive, methylene blue plays a significant role in the fuel industry. It helps reduce corrosion and deposits within engines by preventing the oxidation of fuel components. This action prolongs engine life and enhances performance, offering economic and operational benefits.

By minimizing the formation of gums and varnishes, methylene blue ensures cleaner combustion and more efficient fuel usage, which is crucial for industries reliant on heavy machinery and transportation.

4. Wastewater Treatment Applications

Methylene blue's efficacy in breaking down organic pollutants makes it a valuable asset in wastewater treatment. It acts by adsorbing pollutants and facilitating their removal through chemical reactions. This ability to degrade organic compounds is advantageous in treating industrial effluents, where conventional methods might struggle with complex mixtures.

Its use can lead to significant improvements in water quality, contributing to environmental protection efforts. Compared to other treatment methods, methylene blue offers a cost-effective and efficient solution, although its effectiveness can be influenced by factors such as pollutant concentration and water pH levels.

Methylene blue's versatile properties make it an indispensable component in various industrial applications, from quality control in manufacturing to environmental management. Continued innovation and research are likely to expand its uses and improve its performance, further solidifying its role in industrial processes.

Veterinary Medicine

Methylene blue is a critical therapeutic agent in veterinary medicine, known for its diverse applications in treating various animal conditions. Its effectiveness and versatility make it an invaluable tool for veterinarians managing both emergency and chronic animal health issues.

1. **Treatment of Cyanide Poisoning**

    Cyanide poisoning in animals, particularly in ruminants like cattle and sheep, can occur from ingesting plants like sorghum or certain industrial chemicals. Methylene blue is a proven antidote for this condition. It works by converting methemoglobin to a form that can bind cyanide, facilitating its excretion from the body.

    This treatment is highly effective when administered promptly, significantly improving survival rates. The typical administration involves intravenous injection, providing rapid relief from symptoms such as respiratory distress and neurological impairments. However, the success of methylene blue largely depends on the timing of the intervention and the dose administered.

2. **Prevention of Urinary Tract Infections in Cats**

    In feline medicine, methylene blue is sometimes used to prevent urinary tract infections (UTIs). It acts as a mild antiseptic, reducing bacterial load in the urinary tract. While not a first-line treatment, its use can be beneficial in recurrent cases where conventional treatments have failed.

The administration is usually oral, which helps maintain urinary health by altering the pH and bacterial flora of the urinary tract. However, its use in cats should be approached with caution due to potential side effects and the risk of causing methemoglobinemia if overdosed.

3. **Antidote for Toxicities**

Methylene blue is an effective antidote for several toxicities in pets and livestock. In cases of paracetamol (acetaminophen) overdose, commonly seen in dogs and cats, methylene blue can help reverse methemoglobinemia, a dangerous condition caused by the drug. Similarly, in sheep, methylene blue is used to treat copper toxicity, a condition that can lead to severe liver damage and hemolysis.

The treatment involves administering methylene blue intravenously to reduce methemoglobin levels and restore normal blood function. While effective, these treatments require careful dosing and monitoring to prevent complications.

Ongoing Research and Development

Current research in veterinary medicine is exploring new applications and formulations of methylene blue to enhance its effectiveness and safety. Studies are investigating its potential in treating other toxicities and infections, as well as its role in improving animal recovery post-surgery. Innovations in delivery methods and combination therapies may expand their use in the future, offering more comprehensive solutions for animal health challenges.

Methylene blue's applications in veterinary medicine are diverse and vital, providing critical interventions in both acute and preventative care. As research continues to evolve, its role in veterinary practice is likely to expand, benefiting animal health and welfare across various species.

Health Benefits of the Methylene Blue

Methylene Blue is a synthetic compound that has been around since the late 19th century. Originally developed as a dye, it quickly found its place in the medical world due to its unique properties. Over the years, Methylene Blue has been recognized for its versatility and has been used in various medical applications, ranging from treating certain blood disorders to being a potential cognitive enhancer.

Methylene Blue Health Benefits

1. ***Treatment of Methemoglobinemia***: One of the primary medical uses of Methylene Blue is in the treatment of methemoglobinemia, a condition where hemoglobin is unable to effectively release oxygen to body tissues. Methylene Blue acts as an antidote by converting methemoglobin back to hemoglobin, thereby restoring normal oxygen transport and alleviating symptoms of the condition.
2. ***Cognitive Enhancement***: Recent studies have explored the potential of Methylene Blue as a cognitive enhancer. It is believed to improve mitochondrial function, which is crucial for energy production in brain cells. This enhancement can lead to improved memory retention and cognitive function, making it a promising candidate for addressing age-related cognitive decline.
3. ***Neuroprotective Effects***: Methylene Blue has shown potential neuroprotective properties, which may help in the management of neurodegenerative diseases like Alzheimer's and Parkinson's. It appears to reduce oxidative stress and inflammation, two key factors involved in neuronal damage, thus contributing to the preservation of cognitive health over time.
4. ***Antimicrobial Properties***: The compound also exhibits antimicrobial activity, making it useful in treating certain infections. Its ability to combat pathogens

without causing significant harm to human cells adds to its medicinal value in infection control.
5. ***Mood Stabilization***: Preliminary research suggests that Methylene Blue may have mood-stabilizing effects. It may interact with neurotransmitters in the brain, such as serotonin and dopamine, which play a crucial role in regulating mood. This property could open new avenues for treating mood disorders.

Methylene Blue stands out as a multi-functional therapeutic agent, offering a range of health benefits from treating blood disorders to potentially enhancing cognitive function and providing neuroprotection. Its long history of medical use underscores its importance and continued potential in various health applications.

However, it's crucial to approach its use with caution. As with any therapeutic agent, careful consideration and professional guidance are necessary to ensure safety and efficacy. Further research will help to better understand the full scope of its benefits and any long-term implications of its use.

Disadvantages of the Methylene Blue

While Methylene Blue is a versatile and valuable compound across various fields, it does come with certain disadvantages that are important to consider. However, it's crucial to recognize that the advantages often outweigh these drawbacks, making it a significant tool in scientific and medical applications.

1. **Limited Efficacy in Certain Conditions**

   While Methylene Blue has established effectiveness in treating methemoglobinemia, a condition where hemoglobin is unable to effectively release oxygen to body tissues, its efficacy for a range of other medical conditions, such as cognitive enhancement or various mental health treatments, remains the subject of ongoing research.

   Current studies show promising results regarding its potential benefits in these areas, particularly in enhancing cognitive function and mood stabilization. However, the existing research is not yet conclusive enough to advocate for its widespread use for such purposes, underscoring the necessity for further comprehensive studies to draw definitive conclusions.

2. **Staining and Handling Concerns**

   As a dye, Methylene Blue is known for its intense coloration, which can easily stain skin, clothing, and laboratory equipment. This characteristic necessitates careful handling and the implementation of protective measures, such as the use of gloves and protective eyewear, to prevent unwanted staining.

While this can be viewed as a minor inconvenience in laboratory settings, it is manageable with proper precautions and awareness among the personnel handling the substance. Additionally, educating team members on the correct procedures for handling Methylene Blue can further minimize the risk of accidental staining.

3. **Environmental Impact**

   Although Methylene Blue is utilized in various environmental applications, such as water treatment and dyeing processes, improper disposal or accidental release into water bodies can significantly contribute to water pollution.

   Such environmental concerns highlight the importance of adhering strictly to disposal regulations and environmental guidelines to ensure that Methylene Blue does not negatively impact aquatic life or ecosystems. Furthermore, raising awareness about responsible disposal methods and the potential environmental consequences of improper handling can help mitigate these risks.

4. **Contraindications and Interactions**

   In medical contexts, Methylene Blue can interact with certain medications, particularly antidepressants, which may lead to severe conditions such as serotonin syndrome, a potentially life-threatening condition that arises from excessive levels of serotonin in the brain.

This interaction emphasizes the critical need for cautious use of Methylene Blue and the importance of thorough consultation with healthcare providers before administration. Healthcare professionals should evaluate a patient's complete medication profile and health history to avoid any dangerous interactions that could jeopardize the patient's safety.

5. **Potential Toxicity**

At high concentrations, Methylene Blue has been found to be toxic to certain cell types or organisms, which necessitates controlled and precise application, especially in research environments where cell cultures are involved.

Researchers must carefully calculate dosages and monitor conditions to ensure that Methylene Blue's applications do not inadvertently harm sensitive biological systems. This underscores the importance of protocol adherence and the need for comprehensive training for personnel working with Methylene Blue to minimize any risks associated with its use.

Despite these disadvantages, Methylene Blue remains a cornerstone in sectors such as medicine, biological research, and environmental science. Its ability to act as a staining agent, therapeutic compound, and photosensitizer underscores its multifaceted utility.

By acknowledging and managing the potential downsides, users can harness the significant benefits Methylene Blue offers, contributing to advancements in health, science, and sustainable practices.

Pros and Cons of the Methylene Blue Treatment

The methylene blue treatment has proven to be effective in treating a variety of toxicities and infections in animals. However, like any medication, it also has its drawbacks. In this chapter, we will explore the pros and cons of using methylene blue as a treatment option for pets and livestock.

Pros

The following are some of the advantages of using methylene blue in veterinary medicine:

1. **Proven Effectiveness**

    Methylene Blue has a long-standing reputation for its effectiveness in medical practice, especially in treating methemoglobinemia—a condition wherein the blood loses its ability to carry oxygen efficiently. This condition can be life-threatening, and Methylene Blue serves as a reliable antidote by converting methemoglobin back to functional hemoglobin, rapidly restoring the blood's oxygen-carrying capacity.

Over the decades, its successful application has extended beyond methemoglobinemia to treat other toxicities, further solidifying its track record. The compound's consistent performance in these critical situations underscores its reliability, making it a staple in veterinary practices worldwide.

2. Fast-Acting Nature

One of the most notable attributes of Methylene Blue is its fast-acting mechanism. In cases of severe hypoxia—where oxygen levels in the blood are dangerously low—it can swiftly reverse the condition, often within minutes. This rapid response is crucial in emergency scenarios where time is of the essence.

By quickly restoring proper oxygenation, Methylene Blue not only saves lives but also significantly enhances recovery times for animals experiencing acute illnesses. This immediacy in action allows veterinarians to stabilize patients quickly, paving the way for further treatment and care.

3. Cost-Effectiveness

In addition to its medical benefits, Methylene Blue is also celebrated for its cost-effectiveness. Compared to many other treatments, it is relatively inexpensive, making it an attractive option for veterinary practices of all sizes.

This affordability ensures that even smaller or resource-limited practices can offer high-quality care without imposing undue financial strain on pet owners. The economic accessibility of Methylene Blue allows for broader implementation in routine and emergency veterinary care, ensuring that essential treatment is within reach for all animals in need.

4. Importance in Animal Emergency Cases

The availability and ease of access to Methylene Blue further bolster its importance in veterinary care, particularly in emergency situations. It is widely available and can be easily obtained even in remote or underserved areas, ensuring that veterinarians can respond swiftly to critical cases.

This accessibility is vital in emergencies where every moment counts, allowing for timely intervention that can be the difference between life and death. Its presence as a staple in veterinary medicine cabinets ensures that lifesaving treatment is always at hand.

Methylene Blue's proven effectiveness, rapid action, affordability, and accessibility make it a cornerstone in veterinary medicine. Its ability to quickly reverse life-threatening conditions and its wide availability underscore its significance as a therapeutic agent.

As veterinary practices continue to face a myriad of challenges, Methylene Blue remains a reliable and essential tool, ensuring that animals receive the best possible care in both routine and emergency situations.

Cons

Despite its many benefits, there are also several drawbacks to using methylene blue as a treatment option:

1. **Limited Applications**

    While Methylene Blue is highly effective for certain conditions, its use is not universal. It is primarily employed in treating methemoglobinemia, where it acts to restore the blood's ability to carry oxygen, and in cyanide poisoning, where it serves to counteract the toxic effects. However, it may not be suitable or effective for other illnesses or injuries that do not involve these specific mechanisms.

    This limitation necessitates a thorough diagnosis to ensure that Methylene Blue is the appropriate treatment option for the condition at hand, emphasizing the need for veterinarians to carefully assess each case.

2. **Possible Adverse Reactions**

    As with any medication, Methylene Blue carries the risk of adverse reactions. Animals may experience side effects such as nausea, vomiting, diarrhea, and skin rashes. More severe reactions, though rare, can occur, making it crucial for veterinarians to monitor animals closely following administration.

Prompt identification and management of any adverse effects are essential to mitigate potential harm. This vigilance ensures that treatment with Methylene Blue remains safe and effective, with any complications addressed swiftly.

3. Importance of Proper Dosage

Administering the correct dosage of Methylene Blue is critical to its success as a treatment. An insufficient dose may fail to effectively treat the condition, while an excessive dose can lead to toxicity and additional health issues.

Determining the appropriate dosage requires a comprehensive understanding of the animal's condition and health status, as well as adherence to veterinary guidelines. Veterinarians must exercise precision in dosing to optimize therapeutic outcomes and minimize the risk of complications.

4. Safety Concerns for Certain Animals

Methylene Blue is generally safe for most pets; however, it poses significant risks for animals with a genetic deficiency known as G6PD (glucose-6-phosphate dehydrogenase). In these animals, exposure to Methylene Blue can cause red blood cells to rupture, leading to anemia and other serious health problems.

This condition can affect certain breeds of cats and dogs, necessitating genetic screening or alternative treatments for susceptible animals. Understanding and identifying this risk is crucial for ensuring the safe use of Methylene Blue in veterinary practice.

While there are potential drawbacks to using methylene blue in veterinary medicine, its benefits far outweigh the risks when used correctly.

A Step-by-step Guide to Understanding Methylene Blue

Methylene blue is a medication commonly used in the treatment of a variety of conditions, including urinary tract infections, malaria, and methemoglobinemia. It is also frequently used as a dye during diagnostic procedures.

However, this powerful medication can have serious consequences if misused or taken in excessive amounts. In this guide, we will walk you through the proper use and potential side effects of methylene blue.

Step 1: Educate Yourself on the Proper Usage of Methylene Blue

Methylene Blue is a versatile medication used in various medical treatments. It's essential to understand its proper usage to ensure safety and effectiveness. Below is a detailed guide on how Methylene Blue is used, focusing on administration methods, dosage considerations, and the importance of professional medical guidance.

1. **Administration Methods**
   - *Intravenous Administration*

     For specific medical conditions, such as methemoglobinemia, Methylene Blue is administered intravenously. This method is typically carried out in a hospital setting under the supervision of healthcare professionals. Intravenous administration allows for precise control over the dosage and immediate monitoring of the patient's response, ensuring optimal safety and effectiveness.

   - *Oral Administration*

     Methylene Blue can also be administered orally, particularly for conditions like urinary tract infections. In this form, it is usually available as a tablet. Oral administration allows for more convenient usage but still requires strict adherence to prescribed dosages to prevent potential side effects or complications.

2. **Dosage Considerations**

   The dosage of Methylene Blue can vary significantly based on several factors, including the specific condition being treated, the severity of that condition, and individual patient characteristics such as age, weight, metabolic rate, and overall health status. For instance, pediatric patients may require different dosing compared to adults, and those with pre-existing health issues may need adjustments to avoid complications.

It is crucial to adhere to the dosage guidelines provided by your healthcare provider, as they take into account these important variables. Incorrect dosages can not only lead to ineffective treatment but also result in adverse side effects, which can range from mild to severe.

This emphasizes the critical need for personalized medical advice and careful monitoring during treatment to ensure safety and effectiveness. Always consult with your healthcare professional before making any changes to your medication regimen.

3. Treating Methemoglobinemia

Methemoglobinemia is a condition characterized by the alteration of hemoglobin, the protein in red blood cells responsible for transporting oxygen throughout the body. This alteration leads to a reduced ability of the blood to carry oxygen, which can result in symptoms such as shortness of breath, fatigue, and a bluish tint to the skin. One of the most effective treatments for methemoglobinemia is Methylene Blue, which is commonly administered intravenously in a hospital setting.

Methylene Blue acts by restoring the normal function of hemoglobin, effectively converting methemoglobin back to its oxygen-carrying form. This restoration significantly improves oxygen transport in the blood, alleviating symptoms and enhancing overall oxygen delivery to tissues. Administering Methylene Blue in a hospital ensures that patients receive the correct dosage tailored to their specific needs.

Additionally, it allows healthcare professionals to monitor the patient closely and provide immediate medical intervention if any complications or adverse reactions arise during treatment, ensuring patient safety and optimal outcomes.

4. Addressing Urinary Tract Infections

For urinary tract infections, Methylene Blue may be prescribed in tablet form as an effective treatment option. This medication works by exerting a powerful antiseptic effect on the urinary tract, which helps alleviate symptoms such as burning sensations during urination, frequent urges to urinate, and lower abdominal discomfort. By targeting the source of the infection, Methylene Blue not only alleviates discomfort but also aids in the overall recovery process.

It is crucial for patients to strictly adhere to their physician's instructions regarding the duration and dosage of the medication. Following these guidelines helps ensure a complete resolution of the infection and reduces the risk of recurrence. Additionally, patients should feel encouraged to discuss any side effects or concerns with their healthcare provider to ensure a safe and effective treatment experience.

5. **Importance of Professional Guidance**

Adhering to healthcare professional guidelines when using Methylene Blue is paramount for ensuring safe and effective treatment. Each patient's situation is unique, with varying medical histories, conditions, and responses to medications.

Medical professionals are trained to evaluate these factors and can tailor treatment plans specifically to meet individual needs, optimizing the therapeutic benefits of Methylene Blue. Deviating from prescribed guidelines can not only compromise treatment effectiveness but also pose significant risks to patient safety, potentially leading to adverse reactions or complications. Therefore, it is crucial for patients and caregivers to follow the guidance of healthcare providers to achieve the best possible outcomes.

Methylene Blue is a valuable medication with diverse medical applications. Its proper use, guided by healthcare professionals, is essential for achieving desired medical outcomes while minimizing risks. Patients should always consult their healthcare providers for personalized advice and adhere strictly to prescribed dosage and administration methods.

Step 2: Recognize Potential Side Effects

Understanding the potential side effects of Methylene Blue is crucial for its safe and effective use. Patients need to be vigilant about monitoring symptoms and aware of possible drug interactions. Here, we provide a detailed overview of both common and rare side effects, highlighting the importance of consulting healthcare providers.

Common Side Effects

Methylene Blue can cause several mild to moderate side effects that patients should be aware of:

- *Nausea and Vomiting*: Some individuals may experience gastrointestinal discomfort, including nausea or vomiting, especially shortly after administration.

- ***Dizziness***: Feeling lightheaded or dizzy is a common symptom that may occur as the body adjusts to the medication.
- ***Headaches***: Patients might experience headaches of varying intensity as a side effect.
- ***Diarrhea***: Digestive upset can also manifest as diarrhea, which should be monitored, especially if it is persistent.

These side effects are typically manageable and resolve on their own. However, if they persist or worsen, it is important to seek guidance from a healthcare professional.

Rare and Severe Side Effects

While rare, Methylene Blue can lead to more severe reactions that require immediate medical attention:

- ***Serotonin Syndrome***: This serious condition can occur if Methylene Blue is taken with other medications that increase serotonin levels, particularly SSRIs (Selective Serotonin Reuptake Inhibitors) or MAOIs (Monoamine Oxidase Inhibitors). Symptoms include agitation, confusion, rapid heart rate, and muscle rigidity.
- ***Severe Allergic Reactions***: Though uncommon, severe allergic reactions such as rash, itching, swelling, or difficulty breathing may occur.

If any of these severe symptoms are experienced, it is crucial to seek emergency medical care without delay.

Importance of Monitoring Symptoms

Patients are advised to closely observe their body's response to Methylene Blue. Monitoring helps in the early detection of side effects and ensures timely medical intervention if necessary. Keeping a symptom diary can be helpful for discussing any changes with a healthcare provider.

Drug Interactions and Risks

The risk of adverse effects can increase when Methylene Blue is combined with other medications:

Interactions with SSRIs and MAOIs:

Combining Methylene Blue with selective serotonin reuptake inhibitors (SSRIs) or monoamine oxidase inhibitors (MAOIs) can lead to a substantial increase in serotonin levels in the brain. This elevated serotonin can raise the risk of developing serotonin syndrome, a potentially life-threatening condition characterized by symptoms such as confusion, rapid heart rate, and high blood pressure.

Therefore, it is crucial to engage in careful management and maintain open communication with a healthcare provider before mixing these medications, ensuring that patient safety is prioritized and appropriate monitoring is undertaken.

Other Drug Interactions

It is vital to always keep your healthcare provider informed about all medications, supplements, and herbal products you are currently taking. This transparency helps prevent potential interactions that could lead to adverse effects or reduce the effectiveness of your treatment.

Your healthcare provider can then assess the safety and compatibility of your regimen, adjusting dosages or suggesting alternatives as necessary to enhance your overall health and well-being.

Being informed about the potential side effects of Methylene Blue and its interactions is vital for ensuring patient safety. Patients should maintain open communication with their healthcare providers, promptly report any unusual symptoms, and seek medical attention for severe reactions. This proactive approach helps maximize the therapeutic benefits of Methylene Blue while minimizing risks.

Step 3: Implement Safety Precautions

Ensuring the safe use of Methylene Blue involves taking important precautions before and during treatment. Patients should be well-informed and proactive in communicating with their healthcare providers to minimize risks and enhance the effectiveness of the medication. Below, we outline key safety measures to consider.

1. **Disclosure of Medical History**

   Importance of Sharing Medical Background

   Before initiating treatment with Methylene Blue, it's crucial to provide your healthcare provider with a comprehensive medical history. This includes:

   - <u>Existing Medical Conditions</u>: Disclose any chronic or acute illnesses, such as liver or kidney issues, which may affect how your body processes the medication.
   - <u>Allergies</u>: Inform your doctor about any known drug allergies to prevent adverse reactions.

2. **Medication and Supplement Transparency**

   Discussing Current Medications

   An essential part of safety precautions is discussing all medications, supplements, and herbal products currently being taken. Methylene Blue can interact with various substances, potentially altering its efficacy or causing harmful side effects.

   <u>Potential Drug Interactions</u>: Methylene Blue may interact with antidepressants like SSRIs and MAOIs, increasing the risk of serotonin syndrome. It also can affect the action of other medications, requiring dosage adjustments or substitutions.

3. **Special Considerations for Pregnant or Breastfeeding Individuals**

Assessing Risks and Benefits

Pregnant or breastfeeding individuals need to have detailed discussions with their healthcare providers regarding the use of Methylene Blue:

- *Potential Risks*: The medication may pose risks to the developing fetus or nursing infant, including potential developmental issues or adverse reactions. It's crucial for healthcare providers to conduct a thorough evaluation of the individual circumstances, taking into account the mother's health condition, the specific medication being prescribed, and the stage of pregnancy or breastfeeding. This careful assessment helps determine whether the benefits of the medication outweigh the potential dangers it may present to the child.
- *Alternative Treatments*: If the identified risks are deemed significant, healthcare professionals may recommend exploring alternative therapies. These alternatives could include non-pharmacological approaches such as physical therapy, dietary adjustments, or holistic treatments. The primary goal is to ensure the safety and well-being of both mother and child

while effectively managing the mother's health condition.

4. **Role of Healthcare Providers**

   Personalized Medical Advice

   Your healthcare provider plays a vital role in determining the safety and suitability of Methylene Blue for your specific situation. They can:

   - *Assess Individual Risks*: It's crucial to thoroughly evaluate personal health factors, including medical history, lifestyle choices, and existing conditions, as well as any current medications being taken. This comprehensive assessment helps create personalized advice and treatment plans that are well-suited to the individual's unique health profile and needs.
   - *Monitor Treatment Progress*: Conducting regular check-ins is essential for tracking the effectiveness of the treatment regimen. These evaluations enable healthcare providers to make informed adjustments in dosage or modify the treatment strategy based on the patient's response to the medication and any side effects they may be experiencing. This proactive approach ensures optimal management of the patient's health and enhances overall treatment outcomes.

Implementing safety precautions is a fundamental step in using Methylene Blue effectively and safely. By openly communicating with healthcare providers and following their guidance, patients can significantly reduce risks and ensure the best possible treatment outcomes. Always prioritize personalized advice when considering Methylene Blue, particularly if you have special health considerations or are pregnant or breastfeeding.

Step 4: Monitor Your Health

When undergoing treatment with Methylene Blue, diligent health monitoring is crucial to ensure both the effectiveness of the medication and the safety of the patient. Here's a comprehensive guide on what monitoring entails and why it's important.

1. **Importance of Regular Monitoring**

    Regular monitoring by healthcare providers is essential during Methylene Blue treatment for several reasons:

    - *Effectiveness*: Continuous assessments play a crucial role in evaluating the medication's performance by regularly determining whether it is achieving the desired outcomes in treating the underlying condition. This ongoing evaluation allows healthcare providers to make necessary adjustments to the treatment plan,

ensuring that patients receive the most effective care tailored to their specific needs.
- **Safety**: Monitoring is essential for patient safety, as it helps identify any adverse effects early on, allowing healthcare professionals to manage these issues promptly and appropriately. By closely observing patients for any side effects or unexpected reactions, clinicians can make informed decisions about treatment modifications, ensuring that the benefits of the medication outweigh any potential risks.

2. **Types of Monitoring**

    Blood Tests

    - <u>Purpose</u>: Blood tests are frequently conducted to monitor the levels of Methylene Blue in the body, which is a vital step in assessing its overall impact on various blood components, particularly red blood cells. These tests help ensure that the Methylene Blue levels remain within a safe and effective range, which is crucial for preventing any potential side effects and for evaluating the efficacy of the treatment.
    - <u>Frequency</u>: The frequency of these tests varies significantly based on the specific condition being treated and the patient's individual

response to therapy. For instance, patients undergoing intensive treatment may require more frequent evaluations to closely monitor their blood parameters, whereas others might only need tests periodically. This personalized approach helps healthcare providers make informed decisions about ongoing treatment and any necessary adjustments based on the test results.

3. **Physical Assessments**
   - *Regular Check-Ups*: Routine physical assessments are crucial as they offer healthcare providers valuable insights into the patient's response to medication. These check-ups allow for monitoring how well the patient is tolerating the treatment, enabling providers to identify any potential side effects or adverse reactions. Additionally, these assessments can reveal any physical changes, such as weight fluctuations or changes in overall health status, which can inform adjustments to the treatment plan.
   - *Vital Signs Monitoring*: Regularly checking vital signs, including blood pressure, heart rate, respiratory rate, and temperature, is essential for early detection of complications. Monitoring these signs can help healthcare providers spot any concerning trends that may indicate a

problem, such as hypertension or arrhythmias. By keeping a close eye on vital signs, clinicians can intervene promptly, ensuring the patient's safety and well-being throughout their treatment journey.

4. **Reporting Changes and Symptoms**

   Prompt Communication

   - *New Symptoms*: It is crucial for patients and caregivers to report any new symptoms or significant changes in the patient's condition to healthcare providers as soon as possible. This includes not only physical symptoms, such as unexplained pain, fatigue, or fever, but also changes in mood or behavior, such as increased anxiety, depression, or irritability. Prompt reporting can help healthcare professionals assess the situation accurately and adjust treatment plans as needed to ensure the patient's well-being.
   - *Adverse Reactions*: Timely reporting of any side effects experienced by the patient can be instrumental in preventing more serious complications. Early identification of adverse reactions enables healthcare providers to implement interventions, such as adjusting medication dosages, switching to alternative

treatments, or providing supportive therapies. This proactive approach can significantly improve patient outcomes and enhance overall safety during treatment.

5. Adjusting Treatment Plans

Role of Regular Check-Ups

- *Treatment Adjustments*: Based on the monitoring results, healthcare providers may adjust the dosage or frequency of Methylene Blue to optimize treatment outcomes. This process involves careful assessment of the patient's response to the medication, including any side effects or improvements in their condition. By tailoring the treatment plan to the individual's needs, healthcare professionals aim to enhance efficacy and minimize any adverse reactions, ensuring a more personalized approach to care.
- *Alternative Therapies*: If Methylene Blue is not well-tolerated or effective, healthcare providers might consider alternative treatments. These alternatives could include other medications, lifestyle changes, or complementary therapies that align with the patient's overall health goals. By exploring various options, healthcare providers can work with patients to find the

most suitable and effective treatment strategy, ultimately improving their quality of life and health outcomes.

Monitoring your health while using Methylene Blue is a critical component of safe and effective treatment. Regular check-ups, blood tests, and prompt communication with healthcare providers ensure that the medication is beneficial and minimizes risks. By staying vigilant and responsive to changes in health, patients can contribute significantly to the success of their treatment with Methylene Blue.

Step 5: Understand Long-term Use Implications

When Methylene Blue is required for extended periods, it's crucial for patients to comprehend the long-term implications and maintain proactive communication with their healthcare providers. Here, we delve into the key aspects of managing long-term treatment effectively.

1. **Importance of Regular Follow-ups**

   Continuous Management

   - *Regular Check-ins*: Frequent follow-ups with healthcare providers play a crucial role in monitoring the medication's impact over time. These appointments not only help in assessing the therapeutic benefits but also allow for a thorough examination of any adverse effects that might develop. During these check-ins, healthcare providers can discuss any changes in symptoms, side effects, and overall health, ensuring that the patient receives the most appropriate care tailored to their specific needs.

- *Treatment Evaluation*: Routine evaluations are vital to ensure that the treatment remains effective over the long term. These assessments involve a comprehensive review of the treatment plan, enabling healthcare providers to identify any areas that may require adjustments. By regularly analyzing the patient's progress, healthcare professionals can make timely modifications to the therapeutic approach, such as altering dosages, switching medications, or incorporating additional therapies, thereby optimizing the overall treatment experience for the patient.

2. **Managing Ongoing Treatment**

Dosage Adjustments

- *Personalized Dosing*: Long-term use of medications like Methylene Blue may necessitate adjustments in dosage over time to maintain their effectiveness and minimize potential side effects. Healthcare providers play a crucial role in this process, as they can carefully monitor the patient's evolving needs and responses to the treatment. By conducting regular assessments and open conversations about any changes in symptoms or side effects, providers can tailor the dosing regimen to ensure optimal therapeutic outcomes.

- *Therapeutic Monitoring*: Continuous monitoring of therapeutic levels of Methylene Blue is essential in determining the appropriateness of the current dosage. This involves regular blood tests and evaluations to assess whether the levels are within the desired therapeutic range. Such monitoring helps healthcare providers make informed decisions about dosage modifications, ensuring that patients receive the most effective treatment while minimizing the risk of adverse effects. This proactive approach contributes to a more effective and personalized treatment plan.

3. **Potential Cumulative Side Effects**

Awareness and Reporting

- *Cumulative Effects*: As treatment progresses, patients may begin to experience cumulative side effects that were not noticeable at the start of their therapy. These effects can manifest in various ways, such as prolonged nausea that disrupts daily activities, persistent fatigue that affects energy levels and overall quality of life, or fluctuations in mood that could impact relationships and emotional well-being. It is vital for patients to monitor these changes closely and report any concerning symptoms to their healthcare providers immediately, as this allows for timely interventions and adjustments to the treatment plan.

- *Long-term Safety*: Gaining a thorough understanding of which side effects may persist or even worsen with long-term use of medication is crucial for patient safety and well-being. This knowledge empowers patients to make informed decisions about their treatment options. Engaging in continuous and open dialogue with healthcare professionals allows for effective management of these side effects, ensuring that patients receive the necessary support and care throughout their treatment journey. Regular follow-ups can help identify any emerging issues early on, leading to better health outcomes.

4. **Role of Healthcare Providers**

Continuous Monitoring

- *Health Assessments*: Through routine labs and comprehensive physical assessments, healthcare providers can effectively monitor and track any changes in the patient's condition that might be attributable to long-term medication use. These assessments often include blood tests, imaging studies, and detailed evaluations of vital signs, allowing for a thorough understanding of how medications are impacting the patient's overall health.
- *Proactive Adjustments*: By utilizing ongoing assessments, healthcare providers can make informed decisions regarding the management of a patient's medication regimen. This may involve carefully evaluating the effectiveness of the current medications, considering potential side effects, and determining whether to continue, adjust dosages, or switch to alternative treatments. This proactive approach ensures that the patient's treatment plan remains aligned with their evolving health needs.

5. **Communication and Safety**

Engaging in Open Dialogue

- *Patient-Provider Communication*: Maintaining open lines of communication with your healthcare provider is absolutely vital for successful health outcomes. This ongoing dialogue ensures that any concerns, questions, or changes in your health status are addressed promptly and thoroughly. By fostering a supportive relationship with your provider, you contribute to a safer and more effective treatment process, which ultimately enhances your overall well-being and recovery.

- *Informed Decisions*: Being well-informed about the long-term implications of Methylene Blue is crucial for patients. Understanding how this treatment works and its potential effects enables patients to actively engage and collaborate with their healthcare team. This partnership empowers individuals to make educated decisions regarding their treatment plan, ensuring it aligns with their health goals and needs, and ultimately leading to better management of their condition.

Understanding the implications of long-term use of Methylene Blue is essential for maximizing treatment benefits while minimizing risks. Regular follow-ups, effective communication, and continuous monitoring are the cornerstones of successful long-term therapy. By actively engaging with healthcare providers and staying informed about potential side effects, patients can ensure the safe and effective use of Methylene Blue over time.

Step 6: Know When to Seek Help

Understanding when to seek medical assistance during Methylene Blue treatment is vital for ensuring safety and preventing complications. This guide provides essential information on identifying severe reactions and preparing for emergencies.

1. **Recognizing Symptoms of Overdose or Severe Reactions**

   Key Symptoms to Monitor

   - *Severe Dizziness*: If you experience an intense feeling of spinning or a sudden loss of balance that is unusual for you, it could indicate a potential overdose or an adverse reaction to the medication. This sensation might be accompanied by nausea or a feeling of disorientation, and it is important to seek medical advice if it persists.
   - *Shortness of Breath*: Experiencing difficulty breathing or a sensation that you cannot catch your breath is a serious symptom that requires immediate attention. It may be accompanied by a tight feeling in the chest or wheezing, which can indicate a severe allergic reaction or other respiratory issues that need prompt evaluation.

- *Rapid Heartbeat*: An unusually fast heartbeat, especially if it occurs without any exertion or stress, can be a concerning sign of a severe reaction to the medication. This tachycardia may be felt as palpitations or a racing sensation in the chest and should be discussed with a healthcare provider to rule out any underlying issues.

2. **Importance of Immediate Medical Attention**

Acting Quickly

- *Emergency Situations*: In the event of an overdose or severe adverse reaction, a rapid and coordinated response is absolutely critical. Every second counts, as delaying treatment can lead to serious complications, some of which may be life-threatening. It's essential for bystanders and first responders to recognize the signs of an overdose, such as confusion, difficulty breathing, or loss of consciousness, and to act swiftly by calling emergency services and providing immediate assistance.
- *Medical Intervention*: Healthcare providers are equipped to administer a range of appropriate treatments that can effectively counteract the effects of the overdose or adverse reaction. This may include administering antidotes, providing

oxygen, or performing other life-saving procedures. The goal is to minimize potential harm and stabilize the patient as quickly as possible. Additionally, healthcare professionals will monitor the patient closely for any further complications, ensuring comprehensive care throughout the recovery process.

3. Preparedness and Emergency Contacts

Being Ready

- *Emergency Contact Information*: It's crucial to keep a comprehensive list of emergency contacts easily accessible. This list should include your healthcare provider, local emergency services like police and fire departments, and a trusted friend or family member who can assist in an emergency. Make sure to update this list regularly, including their phone numbers and any important details that emergency personnel might need to know about your situation.
- *Access to Medical Records*: Having your medical history and current medication list readily available is essential in emergencies. This information allows emergency responders to understand your health background and any specific medical conditions you may have.

Consider keeping a printed copy of your medical records, along with allergies, previous surgeries, and current medications, in a visible location or on your phone. This can significantly improve the quality of care you receive during critical situations.

4. Educating Yourself and Caregivers

Awareness and Prevention

- *Understanding Risks*: It's crucial to educate yourself about the potential risks associated with Methylene Blue, which include not only common side effects but also serious issues like signs of overdose, such as confusion, difficulty breathing, or unusual skin discoloration. Being informed allows you to recognize these symptoms early and seek medical assistance promptly.
- *Informing Caregivers*: Ensure that family members or caregivers are fully aware of these risks and understand what steps to take in an emergency situation. This includes knowing how to identify signs of an adverse reaction and having a plan for contacting medical professionals or poison control if necessary. Communication and preparedness can make a

significant difference in managing any unexpected health issues.

Knowing when to seek help during Methylene Blue treatment is crucial for managing potential risks effectively. By recognizing symptoms of overdose, acting promptly, and maintaining preparedness, patients can ensure their safety and receive timely medical attention. Staying informed and keeping emergency contacts accessible empowers patients and caregivers to handle emergencies with confidence.

By following these steps, you will be equipped with the knowledge needed to use Methylene Blue safely and effectively. Always prioritize communication with healthcare providers to ensure your treatment aligns with the best medical practices.

Potential Side Effects

Methylene blue can cause several potential side effects, some of which may require medical attention. Here are the key side effects:

1. **Common Side Effects:**

    While methylene blue is an effective treatment for several medical conditions, it can also cause some common side effects. Here's a deeper look into these potential reactions:

- *Arm or Leg Pain*: Patients may experience discomfort or aching in the limbs, which can range from mild to moderate. This type of pain might affect daily activities, especially if it persists. However, it often subsides as the body adjusts to the medication or with over-the-counter pain relief options, such as acetaminophen or ibuprofen.
- *Change in Taste or Loss of Taste*: Alterations in taste perception can occur, leading to a diminished enjoyment of food and beverages. This side effect may result in changes in appetite or dietary preferences. Typically, these changes are temporary and resolve as the treatment progresses.
- *Changes in Skin Color*: Some individuals might notice a bluish tint to their skin, particularly in areas with thin skin or poor circulation. While this can be alarming, it is generally harmless and fades with time once the medication is discontinued.
- *Increased Sweating*: Excessive sweating, especially during the night, can be uncomfortable and disrupt sleep. Patients may need to adjust their clothing or bedding to stay comfortable, and this side effect often diminishes as the body gets used to the drug.

- *Muscle or Joint Pain*: Similar to limb pain, muscle or joint aches can impact mobility and physical activities. They are usually mild and can be managed with rest, hydration, and in some cases, gentle exercise or stretching to alleviate stiffness.
- *Pain at the Infusion Site*: For those receiving methylene blue intravenously, pain or discomfort at the site of injection is possible. This can be managed by alternating infusion sites, applying warm compresses to the area, or using topical anesthetics to reduce irritation.

These side effects are generally mild and temporary, often resolving as the body adapts to methylene blue. Monitoring by healthcare professionals can help mitigate any persistent discomfort and ensure the safe continuation of treatment.

2. **Serious Side Effects**

   Methylene blue, while effective for certain treatments, can also lead to serious side effects that require prompt medical attention. Here's a detailed look at these symptoms:

   Agitation and Confusion

   These symptoms may manifest as restlessness, irritability, or difficulty concentrating, often leading to feelings of frustration and anxiousness. In severe cases, confusion can escalate to a point where it impairs daily functions and decision-making processes, making even simple tasks seem daunting. This necessitates immediate medical evaluation to prevent further complications, as these symptoms can be indicative of underlying health issues that need to be addressed promptly.

Bluish-colored Lips, Fingernails, or Palms

This discoloration, known as cyanosis, is a significant indicator of poor oxygenation in the blood. It can be alarming and may suggest that the body is not receiving adequate oxygen, which is critical for various physiological functions. This situation is a clear sign that medical attention is needed to address possible respiratory or circulatory issues, ensuring that the oxygen supply to vital organs is restored effectively.

Chest Tightness and Difficulty Breathing

These respiratory symptoms can range from mild discomfort to severe breathing difficulties, potentially causing panic and distress. They may indicate an allergic reaction to certain substances or other serious conditions, including asthma or pulmonary embolism.

Urgent medical intervention is critical in such cases to prevent life-threatening scenarios and to ensure that the patient receives appropriate treatment to alleviate these symptoms.

Fast Heartbeat and Dizziness

A rapid heart rate, known as tachycardia, when combined with dizziness can lead to fainting spells, which can significantly impact mobility and pose serious safety risks. These symptoms may indicate issues with the heart's rhythm or other cardiovascular problems.

Therefore, they should be assessed by a healthcare provider to rule out any serious conditions or underlying causes, ensuring that the individual receives the necessary care to stabilize their heart function and overall health.

Skin Rash, Hives, or Welts

These dermatological reactions can signal an allergic response, particularly to substances like methylene blue. These reactions may be accompanied by itching, swelling, or a burning sensation, which can cause considerable discomfort.

Prompt medical attention is warranted to prevent escalation into a more severe reaction, such as anaphylaxis, which can be life-threatening and requires immediate treatment to ensure the safety of the individual affected.

Overactive Reflexes and Poor Coordination

These neurological symptoms can affect motor skills, balance, and overall coordination, leading to an increased risk of falls or injuries. Individuals may experience difficulty performing everyday tasks that require fine motor skills, which can be frustrating and concerning.

A thorough medical assessment is necessary to determine the underlying cause of these symptoms and to implement appropriate treatment strategies to improve motor function and reduce risks.

Unusual Tiredness or Weakness

Profound fatigue and weakness can significantly impact daily activities and overall quality of life, making even simple tasks feel overwhelming. These symptoms might indicate underlying systemic issues, such as anemia, chronic fatigue syndrome, or other medical conditions.

It is crucial that these symptoms are evaluated by a healthcare professional to identify the root cause and to implement a treatment plan that addresses the specific needs of the individual, ultimately improving their energy levels and well-being.

Each of these serious side effects poses significant health risks and underscores the importance of using methylene blue under close medical supervision. Immediate medical intervention is critical to managing these symptoms effectively and ensuring patient safety.

3. **Overdose Symptoms**

   Experiencing an overdose of methylene blue can lead to a series of alarming symptoms that necessitate immediate medical attention. Here's a closer look at these symptoms:

   - *Enlarged Pupils and Blurred Vision*: Overdose can cause the pupils to dilate excessively, leading to sensitivity to light and blurred vision. This can interfere with everyday tasks such as reading or driving and may indicate central nervous system involvement, requiring urgent evaluation by a healthcare professional.
   - *Blue Staining of Urine, Skin, and Mucous Membranes*: A distinctive sign of overdose, this blue discoloration can be visually striking and indicates excessive accumulation of methylene blue in the body. While it may seem benign, it

highlights the need for medical intervention to prevent further complications.

- ***Nausea and Vomiting***: These gastrointestinal symptoms are common in drug overdoses and can lead to dehydration and electrolyte imbalances if persistent. They can severely impact a patient's ability to maintain adequate nutrition and hydration, demanding prompt treatment to manage these effects.
- ***Rapid Shallow Breathing***: This symptom suggests respiratory distress, which can limit oxygen intake and affect organ function. Rapid shallow breathing is a serious condition that can escalate quickly, underscoring the importance of emergency medical care to stabilize breathing and support respiratory function.
- ***Shakiness and Tingling Sensations***: These neurological symptoms can cause discomfort and impair fine motor skills, affecting the ability to perform daily activities. Such signs of nervous system involvement require immediate medical assessment to prevent long-term damage and ensure appropriate management.

Overall, these overdose symptoms not only disrupt normal functioning but also pose significant health risks. Immediate medical intervention is crucial to mitigate these effects, prevent further complications, and ensure patient safety during recovery.

Contraindications and Precautions

Certain conditions and scenarios necessitate caution or avoidance of methylene blue. Understanding these contraindications can prevent adverse effects and ensure safer use.

Contraindications

Methylene blue presents specific contraindications that necessitate careful consideration before use. Understanding these contraindications helps prevent serious adverse effects and ensures safer handling of the compound.

1. *Hypersensitivity to Methylene Blue*

    Individuals with a known hypersensitivity to methylene blue or any of its components should avoid using it, as it can trigger allergic reactions. Such reactions may range from mild skin rashes to more severe manifestations like hives or anaphylaxis, which is a life-threatening condition requiring immediate medical attention. The risk of hypersensitivity underscores the importance of allergy testing or reviewing patient history for any prior allergic episodes related to methylene blue.

2. Glucose-6-Phosphate Dehydrogenase (G6PD) Deficiency

G6PD deficiency is a genetic condition that affects the red blood cells, making them more susceptible to breaking down under certain stressors, including specific medications. Methylene blue is contraindicated in patients with this deficiency because it can induce hemolytic anemia—a condition where red blood cells are destroyed faster than they can be produced. This risk arises because methylene blue can exacerbate oxidative stress in cells, leading to their premature destruction. Therefore, individuals with G6PD deficiency require alternative treatments that do not elevate the risk of hemolysis.

3. Pregnant and Breastfeeding Women

The use of methylene blue during pregnancy and breastfeeding is generally discouraged unless deemed absolutely necessary by a healthcare provider. The compound's ability to cross the placental barrier and its excretion into breast milk raise concerns about potential adverse effects on fetal and neonatal development.

In pregnancy, methylene blue could pose risks such as embryotoxicity or fetotoxicity, affecting the growth and health of the fetus. During breastfeeding, there is a possibility of methylene blue affecting an infant's health and development through breast milk. Hence, any consideration for its use in these circumstances should always involve a thorough risk-benefit analysis conducted by a healthcare professional.

In summary, understanding these contraindications is vital for the safe use of methylene blue. It highlights the need for thorough patient evaluation and the importance of seeking medical advice to determine the appropriateness of methylene blue in these sensitive conditions.

Precautions

When considering the use of methylene blue, it is crucial to be aware of certain precautions, especially for individuals with specific medical conditions or those taking particular medications. Below are the key points that outline these precautions in detail:

1. *Renal Insufficiency*
   - *Importance of Kidney Function*: Methylene blue is primarily excreted through the kidneys. In individuals with normal renal function, it is efficiently processed and eliminated from the body.
   - *Risks for Impaired Renal Function*: For those with renal insufficiency, the excretion process can be significantly hindered. This may lead to

an accumulation of methylene blue in the body, potentially causing toxicity or adverse effects.
- *Recommendations*: Patients with compromised kidney function should use methylene blue under strict medical guidance. Regular monitoring of kidney function and methylene blue levels might be necessary to prevent potential complications.

2. History of Serotonin Syndrome and Use of Serotonergic Drugs

- *Understanding Serotonin Syndrome*: This is a potentially life-threatening condition caused by an excess of serotonin in the central nervous system. Symptoms can range from mild (shivering and diarrhea) to severe (muscle rigidity, fever, and seizures).
- *Interaction with Serotonergic Drugs*: Methylene blue has monoamine oxidase inhibitor (MAOI) properties, which can increase serotonin levels. When combined with other serotonergic drugs (such as certain antidepressants), it can elevate the risk of developing serotonin syndrome.
- *Medical Supervision*: Individuals with a history of serotonin syndrome or those currently on serotonergic medications should only use methylene blue under careful medical supervision. Doctors may adjust

dosages, suggest alternative treatments, or implement additional safety measures to mitigate risks.

3. **General Recommendations**
- *Consultation with Healthcare Providers*: It is essential for individuals considering methylene blue therapy to consult with healthcare professionals to assess their overall health condition and medication regimen.
- *Monitoring and Support*: Continuous monitoring by healthcare providers can help detect early signs of adverse reactions, ensuring timely intervention and adjustment of treatment protocols.

By understanding and adhering to these precautions, patients and healthcare providers can work together to safely incorporate methylene blue into treatment plans when appropriate.

Guidelines for Safe Usage

Adhering to best practices for safe handling and administration of methylene blue can significantly mitigate risks.

1. **Dosage and Administration**

   It is crucial to follow prescribed dosages meticulously, as exceeding the recommended amounts can significantly increase the risk of side effects, which may range from mild to severe depending on the individual. Methylene blue should be administered strictly under the guidance of a qualified healthcare professional, particularly in therapeutic contexts where precise dosing is essential for efficacy and safety.

Ensure that you discuss any other medications or health conditions with your healthcare provider to avoid potential interactions or complications. Regular monitoring may also be necessary to assess the drug's effectiveness and adjust the dosage as needed.

2. **Monitoring and Evaluation**

Regular monitoring for side effects and interactions is crucial for ensuring patient safety and the effectiveness of the treatment. It is essential to keep a detailed record of any symptoms that arise during use, noting their onset, duration, and severity. This information can provide valuable insights into how the medication is affecting the body.

Additionally, it's important to communicate these observations promptly to a healthcare provider, as they can determine if adjustments to the treatment plan are necessary or if further investigation is required to address any concerning symptoms. Maintaining open lines of communication with your healthcare team is key to achieving the best possible outcomes.

3. **Handling and Storage**

   It is crucial to store methylene blue in a cool, dry place, ensuring that it is kept away from direct sunlight and any sources of heat to maintain its stability and effectiveness. Ideally, use an airtight container to minimize exposure to moisture and contaminants. When handling methylene blue, always use appropriate personal protective equipment, such as gloves and safety goggles, to protect your skin and eyes from potential staining or irritation.

   Additionally, ensure that you are in a well-ventilated area to avoid inhaling any dust or vapors that may be released during the handling process. Take care to avoid accidental ingestion by keeping the compound out of reach of children and pets, and always wash your hands thoroughly after handling it.

Understanding the safety and side effects of methylene blue, along with its contraindications, is essential for minimizing risks. By following safe usage guidelines and consulting with professionals when necessary, you can ensure a careful approach to its use.

Conclusion

Methylene Blue, a compound with a rich history and diverse application spectrum, has captured the interest of professionals across numerous fields, from medicine to biology and beyond. As we conclude this guide, it is essential to encapsulate the multifaceted nature of Methylene Blue, analyzing its many uses, benefits, disadvantages, and the inherent pros and cons associated with its application.

Historically, Methylene Blue has been primarily recognized for its role in the medical field. Initially used as a treatment for malaria, it has since evolved into a versatile therapeutic agent. Its uses include acting as an antidote for specific poisonings and treating methemoglobinemia, a condition where hemoglobin's ability to release oxygen to body tissues is impaired. Moreover, its potential in neuroprotective therapies showcases its evolving role in experimental treatments for neurodegenerative diseases such as Alzheimer's.

In laboratory settings, Methylene Blue is invaluable. It acts as a vital stain in biology, allowing for the visualization of cellular structures through microscopy. Its ability to bind to nucleic acids makes it a staple in molecular biology, particularly in gel electrophoresis, where it aids in the visualization of DNA.

The compound's benefits are substantial, driven by its multifaceted applications. In clinical scenarios, Methylene Blue's ability to act as a reducing agent and antioxidant underpins its therapeutic potential. These properties are crucial in mitigating the effects of oxidative stress and cellular damage, which are implicated in various diseases. In diagnostic settings, its use as a dye aids in the delineation of tissues, enhancing the precision of surgical procedures and diagnostic accuracy. Furthermore, its application in scientific research facilitates a deeper understanding of cellular processes, contributing to advancements in molecular and cellular biology.

However, alongside these benefits, it is imperative to consider the disadvantages and limitations associated with Methylene Blue. One of the primary concerns is its potential side effects when used in medical treatments. Common adverse reactions may include nausea, vomiting, and dizziness, while more severe reactions, such as serotonin syndrome, can occur, particularly when used concomitantly with other serotonergic drugs. Therefore, medical oversight is crucial when administering Methylene Blue to mitigate these risks.

Moreover, the compound's use is not without its challenges in scientific contexts. Its staining properties, while beneficial, can sometimes lead to nonspecific binding, complicating the interpretation of results. Additionally, in therapeutic contexts, the precise dosing and long-term effects require thorough investigation to ensure safety and efficacy.

Balancing the pros and cons, Methylene Blue stands out as a compound of significant potential. Its capacity to improve clinical outcomes, facilitate scientific discovery, and contribute to technological advancements underscores its value. However, its application must be approached with caution, emphasizing the critical role of healthcare professionals in guiding its use. Consulting with medical experts ensures that its benefits can be harnessed effectively while minimizing potential risks.

In terms of its broader significance, the compound's utility extends beyond the confines of individual applications. It serves as a testament to the power of interdisciplinary collaboration, bridging the gap between chemistry, biology, and medicine. This synergy fosters innovation, driving forward the development of novel therapies and diagnostic techniques.

The future of Methylene Blue is undoubtedly promising, with ongoing research likely to unveil new applications and insights. Its role in experimental treatments for psychiatric and neurological conditions, as well as its potential to enhance memory and cognitive functions, are areas of active exploration. As research progresses, a deeper understanding of its mechanisms of action will likely refine and expand its applications, further solidifying its place in various scientific and medical fields.

In conclusion, Methylene Blue is a compound that embodies both potential and complexity. Its diverse applications across multiple domains highlight its utility and importance. However, careful consideration of its advantages and disadvantages is essential to maximize its benefits while minimizing risks. As such, its use must be guided by healthcare professionals who can provide tailored advice and ensure safe application. By maintaining a balanced perspective and fostering continued research and collaboration, Methylene Blue can continue to contribute to advancements in science and medicine, ultimately enhancing our understanding and treatment of various conditions.

FAQs

What is Methylene Blue and what are its primary uses?

Methylene Blue is a synthetic dye with a wide range of applications. Initially used as a textile dye, it is now commonly employed in scientific research as a staining agent, in medical treatments for certain conditions like methemoglobinemia, and in environmental science for applications such as solar energy conversion and wastewater treatment.

Is Methylene Blue safe to use, and what precautions should I take?

Methylene Blue is generally considered safe when used appropriately. However, it is essential to handle it with care, following safety guidelines to avoid potential side effects such as skin irritation or allergic reactions. In medical contexts, it should only be used under professional guidance due to possible contraindications and side effects.

How is Methylene Blue used in medical treatments?

Medically, Methylene Blue is predominantly used to treat methemoglobinemia, a condition that affects oxygen delivery in the body. It acts as an antidote by converting methemoglobin back to hemoglobin, thus restoring normal oxygen transport. Its potential roles in neurology and psychiatry are still under research.

Can Methylene Blue be used for cognitive enhancement or mental health treatments?

Research into Methylene Blue's effects on cognitive function and mental health is ongoing. Some studies suggest potential benefits, but more clinical trials are needed to fully understand its safety and efficacy in these areas. It should not be used for these purposes without professional guidance.

What role does Methylene Blue play in biological research?

In biological research, Methylene Blue is used as a staining agent to help visualize cellular structures under a microscope. It is also employed in studies related to mitochondria and cellular respiration due to its ability to function as an electron carrier in biological systems.

Are there any environmental applications for Methylene Blue?

Yes, Methylene Blue is used in environmental science, particularly in the study of solar energy conversion and wastewater treatment. Its properties as a photosensitizer make it valuable for developing sustainable environmental practices.

What are the common misconceptions about Methylene Blue?

A common misconception is that Methylene Blue is solely a dye with no scientific relevance. In reality, it has diverse applications across various fields, including medicine and environmental science. Additionally, while it shows potential in some areas, its use should be guided by scientific evidence and professional advice.

References and Helpful Links

Pioneering thinker – then and now: Methylene blue – BASF-Magazine Creating Chemistry. (n.d.).
https://www.basf.com/global/en/media/magazine/creatingchemistrystories/2015/pioneer-thinker-then-and-now-methlyene-blue#:~:text=Heinrich%20Caro%2C%20a%20German%20chemist,as%20a%20treatment%20for%20Alzheimer's.

THE PCCA BLOG | Methylene Blue: From textile dye to potential clinical Wonder. (2024, January 29).
https://www.pccarx.com/Blog/methylene-blue-from-textile-dye-to-potential-clinical-wonder#:~:text=The%20history%20of%20methylene%20blue,for%20its%20vibrant%20blue%20color.

Methylene Blue injection. (2024, May 1). Cleveland Clinic.
https://my.clevelandclinic.org/health/drugs/20881-methylene-blue-injection#:~:text=Methylene%20blue%20is%20a%20medication,this%20medication%20is%20Provayblue%C2%AE.

Khanapara, D. B., MD. (n.d.). Methemoglobinemia Treatment & management: approach considerations, initial management, pharmacologic therapy, exchange transfusion, and hyperbaric oxygen.
https://emedicine.medscape.com/article/204178-treatment#:~:text=Patients%20with%20mild%20chronic%20methemoglobinemia,the%20urine%20blue%20in%20color.

Methylene Blue (Intravenous route) side effects - Mayo Clinic. (n.d.). https://www.mayoclinic.org/drugs-supplements/methylene-blue-intravenous-route/side-effects/drg-20064695?p=1

Light and Wellness Co. (n.d.-b). The Ultimate guide to methylene Blue. https://www.lightandwellnessco.com.au/products/the-ultimate-guide-to-methylene-blue

Arias-Ortiz, J., & Vincent, J. (2024b). Administration of methylene blue in septic shock: pros and cons. Critical Care, 28(1). https://doi.org/10.1186/s13054-024-04839-w

www.ingramcontent.com/pod-product-compliance
Lightning Source LLC
LaVergne TN
LVHW012033060526
838201LV00061B/4585